THE LEAN MINDSET

Transform Your Body and Life with Sustainable Weight Loss

Dr. Thomas K. McGlynn

TABLE OF CONTENTS

INTRODUCTION

Greetings, and thank you for your interest in "The Lean Mindset: Transform Your Body and Life with Sustainable Weight Loss." In this book, we will discuss the vital part that one's thinking plays in the process of successfully reaching and sustaining one's weight reduction objectives. The conventional method of losing weight frequently places all of its emphasis on diet and exercise alone, ignoring the significant role that our ideas and attitudes can play in determining how successful we are in this endeavor. This book aims to change that by emphasizing the significance of having a healthy mindset during the process of weight loss.

A synopsis of the book is as follows:

This book is broken up into five parts, and each of those chapters discusses a distinct facet of the process of losing weight. In the first two chapters, we are going to delve into the science behind losing weight as well as understanding your body better. We will discuss the impact that stress and lack of sleep have on our bodies, as well as the part that diet and exercise play in the process of shedding unwanted pounds.

In chapters three through five, we will discuss the fundamental part that our thinking plays in determining whether or not we are successful in losing weight. During this session, we are going to work on recognizing and conquering negative thought patterns, developing a positive and proactive attitude, and setting goals that are within our reach. In the third chapter, we will discuss how to implement a healthy lifestyle, including how to create a healthy meal plan, how to incorporate physical activity into your daily routine, how to better manage stress, and how to get better sleep.

Also, we will concentrate on maintaining our motivation and staying on track, as well as providing the resources that are necessary for our success. In this session, we will cover methods for overcoming setbacks and hurdles, developing a support network, celebrating accomplishments, and keeping tabs on future achievements. A summary of the most important takeaways, words of encouragement for a journey that will last a lifetime, concluding remarks, and suggestions for the next step are included in the book's conclusion. The significance of adopting a lean mentality is a common misconception about weight loss is that it can be reduced to a straightforward calculation of caloric intake vs caloric expenditure. Nevertheless, the reality is a great deal more complicated. Numerous elements, including our genes, the amount of stress we experience, the patterns in which we sleep, and most crucially, our thoughts and attitudes, affect our bodies.

The individual's frame of mind is the single most important factor in the outcome of any attempt to lose weight. When it comes to successfully losing weight and keeping it off, having a positive and proactive attitude, setting attainable objectives, and surrounding yourself with encouraging people can make all the difference. On the other side, negative thought habits and a lack of drive can derail even the most meticulously planned route toward weight loss.

In this book, we will be focusing on the significance of having a lean mindset and giving you the tools and resources, you require to create a positive and proactive attitude. In addition, we will be discussing the value of having a lean mentality. You may improve your body and your life, as well as achieve weight loss that is sustained, by making adjustments to your mentality.

CHAPTER 1

Understanding Your Body

In this chapter, we will investigate the science of losing weight and getting a better knowledge of your body. We will discuss the influence that stress and lack of sleep have on our bodies, as well as the function that nutrition and exercise play in the process of shedding unwanted pounds.

The methodology behind successful weight loss:

The process of losing weight is a complicated one that is affected by several variables, some of which are hereditary, age-related, and hormonal. At its most fundamental level, weight loss is the direct consequence of expending more calories than are taken in. Nevertheless, there is more to it than just calculating calories and limiting the amount of food you consume.

Any disturbance in the body's delicate balance of hormones and chemicals that govern appetite and metabolism might make it difficult to lose weight. Hunger and metabolism are both controlled by hormones. If you understand the science of weight reduction and how your body functions, it will be easier for you to make educated choices about your food and lifestyle that will assist you on your road to a healthier weight.

When we think about losing weight, the assumption that we'll be making is that we'll be losing fat. However, losing weight is a more difficult process than that since not all weight reduction necessarily entails shedding fat. When we cut down on calories, our systems do not immediately begin to rely only on the breakdown of stored fat for fuel. If we lived in a perfect world, our bodies would only be able to burn fat; our abdominal fat would be the first to go, and it would be simple to get the appearance of a fitness model. However, sadly enough, that is not the situation. Let's take a look at the process of losing weight from a scientific point of view so that we may have a better understanding of how to be successful.

If you start a diet and restrict the number of calories you take in, the body will burn fat, but if you allow yourself to get too hungry, it will also destroy lean muscle tissue. If you lose too much lean muscle mass by crash dieting, your metabolic rate will naturally slow down. This is a cruel trick of nature, and it's one of the reasons why crash dieters usually end up regaining the weight they lost. We need to be cautious to avoid this issue, but you should be wary of any fad diet that claims you will lose a significant amount of weight or get results in a short amount of time. This kind of diet is likely robbing you of your future in exchange for the illusion of results in the here and now. Since one motivation for weight reduction is to enhance one's future health, we need to approach weight loss most sustainably and healthfully as possible so that we may achieve our goals.

Whether your metabolism is sluggish or quick, you may lose weight if you know what to do. You probably hear a lot of people talking about how fast their metabolism is, but are you familiar with the meaning of the word "metabolism"?

Metabolism Explained

Keeping yourself alive consumes around seventy percent of the calories you burn off every day (called the Basal Metabolic Rate or BMR). These include things like breathing, blood circulation, maintaining body temperature (creating heat), manufacturing new cells and recycling old ones, regulating hormone levels, brain and nerve function, and performing sedentary activities like sleeping, sitting, or checking your smartphone.

Approximately twenty percent of total energy is used up in more strenuous physical activities, such as going to the train, performing housework, or exercising. You have more influence over this aspect of the situation if you engage in more physical exercise. However, unless you go out for the whole day, it will never be able to compare to the number of calories that are burned just by living.

And lastly, around 10% of your energy is spent digesting the food you eat. Whether you are eating "negative calorie items" like celery, which are supposed to require more calories to digest than they offer, or cupcakes, this won't make a significant difference in your weight loss efforts. However, this does not give you the license to gorge yourself on cupcakes.

Both Metabolism and Physical Activity

This demonstrates that even the act of occupying space demands a significant amount of energy. This is excellent news for those who are trying to lose weight since it indicates that physical activity, despite the fact that it is essential to one's general health, may be seen more as a bonus than as a must for doing so. The typical individual would burn between 2000 and 2400 calories each day without going to the gym, and a vigorous training session may cause them to burn an additional 200 calories (which is 8–10% more than they would burn by just lounging about all day).

In addition, while we are considering the number of calories we have burnt, we should avoid "double dipping." If you take into account the fact that our basal metabolic rate (BMR) causes us to burn approximately 100 calories per hour, this means that even though the treadmill may report that you burned 200 calories in an hour of race walking, you would have burned 100 calories simply by standing there, leaving you with an actual deficit of 100 calories for your effort — much less than the gym would like you to believe!

However, one should not give up hope. Your muscles are more physiologically active than the majority of the other tissues in your body, which means that even while at rest, they continue to burn a greater number of calories. And we're not just talking about the muscles that are visible to the naked eye, like your biceps. Even if you don't lift weights, you have a lot of "skeletal muscle," which refers to the muscles that keep your head and neck in the correct position, support your spine, assist with breathing, and provide you the ability to walk and move around. Exercising helps you preserve the muscle you already have or helps you build more muscle, both of which have a small but positive influence on calorie burning over time. Exercising also prevents your metabolism from slowing down as you get older. However, you shouldn't rely on exercise as your major method for getting rid of doughnuts since it is an excellent way to keep your metabolism healthy.

Fat Loss

Fat Loss Studies have shown that a healthy pace for losing fat is between one and two pounds of fat each week. In ideal circumstances, you may also utilize the rule of thumb that you should be able to burn off 1% of your body weight in the form of fat per week. Therefore, if you weigh 300 pounds, you would have three pounds of fat in your body. At 180 pounds, one pound of fat would be equivalent to 1.8 pounds, and so on.

The accumulation of energy in the form of fat in the body is essential to our long-term survival, especially in times of famine. It is a very effective method due to the fact that one gram of fat contains more than twice as much energy as one gram of carbohydrates. Even a lean adult with a healthy level of physical activity has roughly 130,000 calories stored in their relatively low amount of body fat. That's a lot of preparation for emergency situations.

How Our Bodies Save Fat

When we consume carbohydrates in the form of starches and sugars, our bodies convert these foods into glucose, which is the simplest kind of fuel for our cells to oxidize and burn in order to produce energy. When we consume an excessive number of calories, our systems turn the extra glucose into fatty acids and store them in the form of adipose tissue for future use. Amino acids that are in excess as a result of the amount of protein we ate may be transformed into fatty acids and stored. No matter what form the surplus food energy takes, as long as it is present in our circulation, the fat cells will continue to be untapped and will continue to develop. Insulin is a fundamental signal in the complicated hormonal signaling system that controls not only the removal of excess carbs from circulation but also the suppression of the breakdown of fatty tissue. This system is responsible for both processes. Insulin is one of the main signals. An increase in blood sugar caused by a meal causes the production of insulin. Insulin urges our fat cells to hang on to their energy reserves, while also instructing our muscles and other tissues to absorb and burn the glucose as quickly as possible.

How We Get Rid of Fat

As soon as the amount of glucose that is present in the blood decreases, insulin levels will also decrease, and your body will begin to mobilize energy from the fat cells in your body instead. It is a complicated process that is initiated by a number of hormones and carried out by a system of enzymes and coenzymes. First, the fat cells need to be unlocked, then the fatty acids need to be transported into your cells, and finally, the fatty acids need to be broken down into smaller units so that they can be consumed. It is essential to bear in mind that our fat cells will not release their energy reserves while insulin is present, and hence, the most crucial factor in successful fat reduction is a diet that maintains stable blood sugar levels and places them within a healthy range. This requires abstaining from foods containing sugar, processed carbs, white flour, and a large number of ready-to-eat commercial items. Whole foods, which need more digestive energy to break down, are your diet's greatest friend.

Muscle Loss

If all of the glucose that is readily accessible is used up, as well as the fatty acids that can be released from fat cells in a more controlled manner, the body will shift its focus to other tissues, such as muscle. But it is not something that we want to promote in any way. Crash diets should never be attempted for this same reason. Diets that reduce calorie intake by an excessive amount send our bodies into a state of famine, which destroys our lean muscle mass in addition to our fat stores, which in turn slows down our metabolism. There is a "Goldilocks zone" of calorie restriction that maintains our position in the optimal zone for the metabolism of fat. We need to make sure that our calorie intake stays within the optimal range so that we can promote fat loss without putting the body into famine mode. In addition, we structure our meals around a certain ratio of protein, carbohydrates, and fats in order to promote the maintenance of muscle mass while putting an emphasis on the burning of fat. The optimal proportion of nutrients also enables us to experience satiety and keeps hunger at bay, which is a double win. And if we are not hungry, we are less likely to develop desires for unhealthy foods. Therefore, this is a pretty wonderful location to be in.

Water Weight

The loss of water is another factor that may contribute to the scale displaying a lower number. Both glucose and fat can bind water molecules, while water molecules can also connect themselves to fat and glucose. When we burn these fuels, carbon and water are discharged into the atmosphere as byproducts. We exhale the carbon, which is then converted into CO_2, and we naturally urinate out the water. When you initially begin a diet, you may notice that you lose weight more quickly in the first two weeks. This is due to the fact that excess water that has been locked up in your body is being released while your body's energy supplies are being depleted. This is a wonderful and very unremarkable occurrence. If you indulge in a cheat day or go on a binge when attending a birthday celebration, there is another reason why you can discover that your weight has increased again. Following a binge, the number on the scale will rise more quickly than you may anticipate due to the attachment of water molecules to any additional fat or glycogen that your body stores.

The role of diet and exercise

Diet and exercise have a significant part in the process of losing weight since they are both essential components. Maintaining a nutritious diet will assist you in keeping track of the calories you consume while also supplying your body with the nutrients it needs to perform at its very best. Participating in regular physical exercise may assist raise your metabolism, which in turn leads to increased calorie burning and, ultimately, weight reduction.

It is essential that you choose a diet and fitness program that is suitable for you and your body and stick to it. There is no technique for weight reduction that is universally effective, and a strategy that is successful for one individual may not be effective for another. It is really important to pay attention to your body and discover the optimal level of balance for you.

Developing good habits concerning one's food and level of physical activity is essential for effective weight reduction. Diet and exercise are probably not two terms that appeal to your sense of style. But don't let your attention get consumed by them. A diet is nothing more than consuming food that is both nutritious and low in calories. Increasing one's level of physical activity is the definition of exercise. People who are attempting to lose weight understandably place a lot of emphasis on their food; nevertheless, staying active is also a crucial component of any program designed to aid in weight reduction. When you engage in physical activity, your body must use energy in the form of calories to move, which contributes to the burning of the calories that you take in via the food that you consume.

There are many other types of physical exercise, including shopping, mowing the lawn, gardening, making the bed, and cleaning the home. On the other hand, exercise is a more organized and repeated sort of physical activity that you engage in daily. Whatever you decide to do, make it a habit to do it often. Aim for a minimum of 150 minutes of moderate physical activity or 75 minutes of intense aerobic exercise per week, ideally spaced out over the week. Keep in mind that increasing the amount of physical activity you do may be necessary for you to successfully lose weight and keep it off.

The Effects of Stress and Lack of Sleep

Both the effects of stress and patterns of sleep on one's weight reduction efforts may be considerable. The delicate balance of hormones in the body may be thrown off by persistent stress, making it more difficult to shed unwanted pounds. Additionally, not getting enough sleep may contribute to increased appetite as well as a slowed metabolism, all of which make it much more difficult to lose weight.

It is crucial to look for healthy strategies to handle stress, such as engaging in physical activity, practicing meditation, or seeing a therapist. Getting adequate sleep and developing a regular sleep habit might also aid support your weight reduction quest.

In addition, the first step in the route toward weight loss is to have an awareness of your body and how it functions. You will be able to make educated choices about your health and well-being and set yourself up for success if you understand the science behind losing weight, including the importance of nutrition and exercise, as well as the influence that stress and lack of sleep have.

A sufficient amount of sleep improves your chances of being successful in your attempts to lose weight. If a person was getting between six and eight hours of sleep each night, they had a greater chance of reaching their objective of losing at least ten pounds. According to the findings of the research, reducing stress also helps with weight loss.

It was required of all five hundred people who took part in the research that they shed 10 pounds during the trial.

Every participant was present at the weekly check-ins to record their weight and during the instructional sessions. The presenters at the sessions urged the attendees to cut their caloric intake by at least 500 calories per day, adopt a diet that was low in both fat and sugar, and engage in physical activity for at least 180 minutes each week. Participants were instructed to maintain a diary of their sleep duration, stress levels, and mood during the study. The teachers of the workshop strongly suggested that each participant maintain a food journal.

Persons who slept for more than six hours and maintained a lifestyle with minimal stress were about three-quarters as likely to be successful in losing 10 pounds or more, and they were twice as likely to reach their objectives in comparison to people who slept for six hours or less each night.

Because it alters the hormone levels in the body, lack of sleep usually results in weight gain or makes it more difficult to lose weight via food alone. When leptin levels are low and ghrelin levels are high, it might cause the metabolism to slow down while simultaneously increasing hunger for unhealthy foods.

Getting enough sleep should always be a top priority, whether your goal is to reduce body fat or maintain your fitness level throughout the swimsuit season. Adults should strive to obtain at least seven hours of sleep each night, as recommended by the American Academy of Sleep Medicine. Never underrate the power that a healthy diet and regular exercise can have. Weight reduction programs such as Weight Watchers are successful for many individuals in part because they educate participants to help them make better decisions and urge participants to take personal responsibility for their own health.

Making Lifestyle Changes

Making adjustments to one's way of life Losing weight is a process that calls for making adjustments to one's way of life. It is very necessary to strike a balance between maintaining a nutritious diet, engaging in regular physical activity, learning how to effectively handle stress, and obtaining adequate sleep. Making adjustments to your routine might be difficult at times, but they are essential for attaining and keeping off the weight after it has been lost.

Making incremental improvements and expanding on those wins is one of the most important aspects of any successful strategy. To begin started, try increasing the number of fruits and vegetables in your diet, cutting down on the size of the portions you eat, or adding an exercise that gets you moving into your regular routine. As you become used to these adjustments, you'll be able to make more important adjustments, such as eliminating processed foods and added sugar from your diet or ramping up the intensity of your workout program.

Additionally, it is important to exercise patience and refrain from being disheartened. The process of losing weight is a gradual one, and it takes some time before one can notice the benefits. It's vital to concentrate on the progress you have achieved, rather than the objective you have yet to attain. It might be helpful to maintain your motivation and stay on track to celebrate your tiny triumphs along the road.

The Significance of Having a Good Grasp of Your Own Body: The process of losing weight successfully requires that you have a solid understanding of your own body. You are able to make educated choices about your health and well-being if you have a solid grasp of the science behind losing weight, the importance of nutrition and exercise, and the effects that stress and lack of sleep have. Having this information at your disposal may assist you in establishing a diet and exercise regimen that is not only beneficial to your body but also to your overall health and well-being.

In addition, having a good knowledge of your body may assist you in recognizing patterns and routines that may be preventing you from successfully losing weight. For example, you may find that you tend to overeat when you are anxious or that you don't get enough sleep. You may try to modify these habits once you are aware of them, which will put you in a better position to be successful.

In addition to this, one of the most important aspects of the process of losing weight is being familiar with one's own body. You may put yourself in a position to be successful and accomplish weight reduction that is sustainable if you make well-informed choices about your health and fitness. Keep an eye out for the following chapter, in which we will discuss the vital part that your frame of mind plays in the process of shedding unwanted pounds.

Having Objectives That Are Attainable

The process of losing weight successfully requires that you first establish objectives that are attainable. When it comes to goal-setting, it is essential to focus on making progress rather than achieving perfection. You may help yourself stay motivated and on track by setting goals that are both modest and easy to achieve.

It is also essential to bear in mind that the process of losing weight is one that takes time. It is not reasonable to anticipate that one may shed a considerable quantity of weight in a short period of time. You may help yourself avoid frustration and disappointment by setting objectives that are realistic and within your reach, which will also set you up for long-term success.

Incorporating Healthy Habits

Developing healthy routines that are part of your everyday routine will assist support your efforts to lose weight and maintain a healthy weight. For instance, obtaining enough amounts of sleep, drinking a lot of water, and eating a diet that's well-balanced are all things that may assist in weight reduction and general wellness.

It is also necessary to locate appropriate coping techniques for stress, such as engaging in physical activity, practicing meditation, or seeing a therapist. Getting into the habit of practicing healthy behaviors will help you keep the weight off and set you up for success in the long run.

The Strength That May Be Gained Via Introspection

The process of losing weight involves a significant amount of introspection on your behalf. Spending some time thinking about your routines, actions, and beliefs will assist you in recognizing patterns and routines that may be preventing you from achieving your goal of losing weight. You could, for instance, come to the conclusion that you have the propensity to overeat in times of high stress or that you have unfavorable ideas about the appearance of your body. You may try to modify these habits once you are aware of them, which will put you in a better position to be successful. You may create methods for success as well as an awareness of your own talents and flaws by engaging in some self-reflection.

Keeping One's Motivation

Maintaining one's motivation during the process of weight reduction is a vital component. When you first start a strategy to lose weight and don't see results immediately away, it might be difficult to maintain your dedication to the program. However, it is essential to bear in mind that losing weight is a long process, and that progress may not always be visible on the scale. Keeping this in mind may help keep your expectations realistic.

It is essential to keep one's attention on progress rather than perfection in order to maintain one's motivation. You may help yourself stay motivated and on track by celebrating the little triumphs along the road, such as when you accomplish a goal or when you test out a new healthy meal.

In addition to this, it is very necessary to have a support system in place. You may help yourself remain motivated and on track by surrounding yourself with people who understand your objectives and who can give encouragement and accountability. This might be friends, family, or members of a support group.

The significance of mental attitude

Your frame of mind is one of the most important factors in successful weight reduction. It's possible that the way you think about things like diet, exercise, and your own body can significantly affect how successful you are. For instance, engaging in self-defeating behaviors such as binge eating or missing exercises because you have a pessimistic outlook about your physical appearance is a kind of self-sabotage.

The role of mindset

It is very necessary to develop a constructive and empowered frame of mind. This entails adopting a "growth mentality," in which one is more concerned with making progress and gaining knowledge than with attaining perfection. It also involves shifting your attention away from harsh judgments of yourself and toward acts of self-care and kindness.

Nevertheless, maintaining one's motivation and cultivating a mentality that is optimistic and self-affirming are essential components of the process of weight reduction.

You may put yourself in a position to succeed and accomplish weight reduction that is sustainable if you adopt a growth mindset, keep track of your progress, and surround yourself with people who will encourage you.

The importance of finding the right weight loss plan

The significance of selecting the appropriate weight-loss strategy It is essential to your success to choose the appropriate weight-loss strategy. There is no technique for weight reduction that is universally effective, and a strategy that is successful for one individual may not be effective for another. It is crucial to locate a plan that matches your way of life, tastes, and the specific requirements of your health.

For instance, some individuals may discover that the greatest diet for them is one that is low in carbohydrates, while others may find that they do better with an approach that is more balanced. While some individuals discover that they like and are effective with a regular training program, others may find that they are more comfortable with more casual forms of physical activity.

When selecting a program for weight reduction, it is essential to take into account both your current state of health and any preexisting issues you may have. If you suffer from a medical condition such as diabetes, for instance, you may have to alter the foods you eat in order to make room for your prescribed medicine.

In conclusion, selecting the appropriate strategy for weight reduction is an important step in the process of shedding excess pounds. You may set yourself up for success and accomplish weight reduction that is sustainable if you take the time to choose a plan that is appropriate for you, take into account the requirements of your health, and make adjustments as necessary. In the next chapter, we are going to talk about how important it is to keep track of your progress. Keep an eye out!

CHAPTER 2

Changing Your Mindset

Your frame of mind is a very important factor in the success of your weight reduction quest. If you want to remain motivated, make better decisions, and accomplish what you set out to do, adopting a mentality that is positive and powerful will help.

Taking Care of Oneself and Loving Oneself Involves

A healthy and optimistic frame of mind necessitates the practice of both self-care and self-love. You may build a positive and empowered frame of mind by giving yourself time to participate in things that offer you pleasure and that make you feel good about who you are.

Taking a soothing bath, reading a book, engaging in a yoga practice, or going for a stroll outside in nature are all great examples of activities that fall under the category of self-care. You may also include self-care into your regular schedule by doing things like meditating, keeping a gratitude notebook, or practicing thankfulness at regular intervals throughout the day.

You may create a positive and empowered mentality by practicing self-compassion and putting your attention on your strengths and good attributes and concentrating on what you do well. Try to be kind and patient with yourself, and keep your attention fixed on the progress you've made and the accomplishments you've attained.

Adopting An Attitude of Continuous Improvement

A growth mentality is one that places a greater emphasis on continual improvement and development than it does on attaining perfection. When you adopt a growth mindset, you adopt the concept that you are capable of learning new things and growing as a person. You also adopt the notion that failures and other types of setbacks provide chances for development and progress.

You may create a positive and empowered mentality by putting your attention, rather than on attaining perfection, making progress, and expanding your knowledge. When you are faced with obstacles or failures, rather than obsessing over what went wrong, try to shift your attention to what you can take away from the experience and how it might help you improve in the future.

Reframing Negative Thoughts

Reframing unhelpful ideas Negative thoughts have the potential to slow you down and prevent you from making progress. If you find that you are experiencing negative thoughts, you should make an effort to reinterpret them in a more optimistic way. Think of it this way: rather than saying to yourself, "I'll never be able to lose weight," try saying to yourself, "I may struggle at times, but I'm learning and making progress."

You may create a positive and empowered mentality by changing the way you think about unfavorable situations and events. You may also give it a go to engage in positive self-talk and concentrate on the positive aspects of your personality and character.

There are certain ways in which the psychology of losing weight might work against you, but there are also ways in which it can work for you. In order to go around the obstacle that you are facing, the first thing you will need to do is pinpoint exactly what the obstacle is.

Thinking That Either One Is True or False

All-or-nothing thinking is a cognitive distortion that manifests itself when a person feels as though they must choose between completely adhering to their diet plan or completely deviating from it. If you often feel as though you must choose between the two, you may be experiencing this cognitive distortion.

The word "cognitive distortion" is a term that is used by psychologists to refer to persistent and exaggerated ideas that are not in sync with what is really taking on in the real world. People who are attempting to lose weight but have a mentality of "all or nothing" feel that their weight loss efforts will either be a full success or a total failure depending on the foods they choose to eat.

Studies have demonstrated that a thinking style known as "all-or-nothing" is directly associated with a perceived lack of control over eating as well as difficulty maintaining a healthy weight. This lack of control has been compared by some scholars to the kind of conduct shown by Jekyll and Hyde.

If you engage in thinking that is either all or nothing, you probably find it difficult to go back into a healthy eating habit after indulging in a very little treat. Instead, you are likely to give up on your diet and start binge eating since you have concluded that it is pointless to continue trying to lose weight.

A Poor Self-Image of One's Body

If you want to alter the size and form of your body, you probably aren't happy with how it appears in its present condition, especially if you are attempting to make such changes. There is really nothing wrong with acknowledging that you have the desire to enhance either your health or your attractiveness. But if you have a poor body image, it may be detrimental to both your self-esteem and your ability to make improvements.

A poor body image might be directly linked to low self-worth for some individuals. They can believe that their value is based on factors such as their physique, their form, their size, or the food that they consume.

When attempting to achieve and keep a healthy weight, as well as form and maintain appropriate eating habits, this may be a significant obstacle to success. A poor opinion of one's own physique is associated not only with unhealthy eating practices but also with other difficulties.

People who have painful preoccupations with their weight and form may also have emotions of shame in public, avoidance of activities because of feelings of self-consciousness, and excessive sensations of fatness after eating as a result of their concerns. They may classify foods as "good" or "bad" and place an emphasis on low-calorie foods rather than those that are high in nutrients.

It is not quite apparent if having a poor body image contributes to unhealthy eating or whether unhealthy eating contributes to having a poor body image. It should come as no surprise that having a strong sense of discontent with one's physical appearance may make it difficult to achieve a healthy weight and, more crucially, can be detrimental to one's mental well-being and sense of self-worth.

Depression

Although it is unclear to researchers whether depression leads to weight increase or if it acts as a barrier to weight reduction, many experts feel there is a connection between the two. And even in those who have a healthy weight for their height and build, depression may still cause weight-related complications.

Depression is known to cause a decrease in appetite and subsequent weight loss in certain individuals. According to the findings of several studies, even having the notion of being overweight might enhance a person's level of psychological discomfort and could even contribute to depression.

The symptoms of depression, such as an inability to sleep or extreme exhaustion, might make it more difficult to lose weight. In addition, several antidepressants that are often provided to patients might also cause them to gain weight. It is imperative that you discuss your depressive symptoms with either your primary care physician or a mental health professional. It is far more important to address your mental health than it is to lose weight.

Suggestions for Overcoming Obstacles

Keep a Diary or Journal.

It is not always easy to avoid experiencing stress. You can, however, figure out what causes your stress and make an effort to steer clear of the circumstances and individuals that are detrimental to your progress. Keeping a diary during the procedure might prove to be beneficial. In point of fact, studies have shown that maintaining a diary may increase the effectiveness of weight reduction efforts by a factor of two.

There are several applications for keeping a journal. For instance, you may keep track of the food that you eat by using a notebook. On the other hand, you may utilize it to jot down your ideas and figure out what causes your stress. Make use of the notebook to keep track of any circumstances or meals that may seem like a trigger to you and record your thoughts and feelings about them.

Introduce Moderate Alterations

If you have a mindset that makes it impossible for you to keep to your diet plan, you should give some thought to taking baby steps and establishing short-term objectives.

The first step is to zero in on a single particular healthy modification that is both realistic and reasonable. Remind yourself that the aim is not perfection, but rather that any endeavor to move in the right way is progress that you should be proud of. Perfection is not the goal; rather, the goal is to nudge yourself in the correct direction.

You may decide to go for a stroll every night for the remaining 15 minutes after supper. Make it your mission to zero down on that one objective for the next seven days. If you maintain a diary, each day you should write down some notes regarding the many ways you have been successful in keeping that objective front and center in your mind. And remember to give yourself some credit. Keep in mind that even the smallest of actions is preferable to doing nothing at all.

Taking baby steps might help you avoid making too many changes all at once by easing you into the process. If you take on too much at once, you run the risk of being overwhelmed, which may lead to a loss of motivation. On the other hand, if you are able to bring about a little adjustment with success, you will experience a feeling of fulfillment that will encourage you to go on with your efforts.

Listen to Self-Talk

Do you give the messages that you send to yourself throughout the day the attention they deserve? It's possible that these recurring ideas are becoming an obstacle in the way of your health.

Those who are prone to having a poor body image may discover that they constantly repeat negative messages to themselves about their body at various points throughout the day. Phrases like "I'm so obese" or "I'm so out of shape" might make it more difficult for you to take a step toward a healthier lifestyle when the chance arises, whether you say them out or think them in your brain.

All-or-nothing thinking may also manifest itself via a person's internal monologue or self-talk. You could, for instance, discover that you are too hard on yourself for not meeting the unreasonably high standards or objectives that you have set for yourself.

Take a week or two to listen to your inner conversation. Identify one or two messages that may be fostering a poor self-image and write them down. You may then confront them or replace these messages with a strong mantra. Phrases such as "my body are strong," "I am enough," or "I have come a long way" are mantras that are widely employed to enhance confidence.

Learn Relaxation Techniques

If you can't avoid the people or locations that generate stress, relaxation methods might be a good option for regulating emotions during difficult times.

Scientists have shown that a certain relaxation method, guided imagery, may aid with weight reduction. You can work with a therapist to learn guided imagery, but it's feasible to practice it on your own. If you find that you tend to overeat in times of stress because your emotions are driving you to do so, guided imagery may be the most efficient strategy for helping you lose weight. However, mastering it will take some time.

Prioritize Sleep

Researchers have again and again discovered a connection between poor sleeping habits, increased body fat, and bad eating patterns. Improving one's nighttime routine is perhaps one of the easiest and most relaxing measures that can be taken in the process of overcoming psychological hurdles.

Make your bedroom a haven for sleep by creating a routine that includes going to bed at the same time every night and getting up at the same time every morning. Remove any electrical devices, such as the television, computer, and mobile phone charger, and make as many efforts as you can to lessen the amount of background noise.

You may create a completely black environment in your bedroom by hanging light-blocking curtains or purchasing an affordable sleep mask. Some folks find that turning the temperature down helps them get a more peaceful night's sleep.

Seek Help

Many professionals have received specialized training to address mental health conditions such as depression and anxiety, as well as other problems that may be preventing successful weight reduction. It is possible to locate a behavioral health professional who is experienced in the treatment of the underlying emotional reasons for excessive eating and weight gain.

Your healthcare professional may be able to issue a recommendation. In the event that this is not possible, there are various methods to discover a therapist. The American Psychological Association provides customers with access to a variety of services that may assist them in obtaining the assistance they need, such as a locator service that can be used to identify practitioners in their local region.

Consider utilizing one of the recently established applications or technological tools that may give mental health therapy by text, Skype, or Facetime in the event that your circumstances prohibit you from visiting a behavioral health practitioner in person. These types of treatment services often provide relief at a cost that is far lower than that of traditional face-to-face counseling.

Creating a Positive Environment Around Yourself

You may build a positive and empowered attitude by surrounding yourself with good and supportive people, activities, and settings. This can help you cultivate a positive and empowering perspective. Seek out a support system in the form of friends, family, or a support group that can encourage you and hold you accountable for your progress.

In addition, make an effort to seek out material that is encouraging and uplifting for you, such as books, movies, or podcasts that may help you become more inspired and motivated. Stay away from sources of negativity, such as television news shows that only report on violent and contentious events.

In conclusion, cultivating a positive and empowered attitude requires engaging in self-care and self-love practices, adopting a growth mindset, recasting negative beliefs, and surrounding oneself with positivity. You may reach your weight reduction objectives by adopting these practices, as well as build a good and empowered mentality for yourself in the process.

CHAPTER 3

Implementing a Lean Lifestyle

In this chapter, we will delve into the more tangible parts of putting a lean lifestyle into practice, such as how to make good food choices, how to include physical exercise into your daily routine, and how to develop healthy habits. You will be able to make long-lasting changes to your lifestyle and accomplish your weight reduction objectives if you read this chapter and follow the guidelines and advice that are presented in it.

Picking Nutritious Options from the Menu

Making decisions about meals that are good for you is one of the most crucial aspects of leading a healthy lifestyle. In this subchapter, we will discuss numerous suggestions and techniques for making healthy food choices, such as meal planning, grocery shopping, and dining out. These are all common situations in which people find themselves in need of assistance.

Meal Planning

The process of preparing meals is an essential component of making decisions on the consumption of nutritious foods. It is possible to guarantee that you will consume healthy and well-balanced meals that will help you achieve your weight reduction objectives if you plan your meals in advance.

Making use of a meal calendar is one of the most efficient ways to arrange one's meals. This may make it easier for you to monitor what you eat and ensure that you are eating a range of meals that are both healthy and well-balanced for your body. You will have a backup plan in the form of pre-planned meals if you plan your meals in advance, which will help you resist the temptation of eating items that are bad for you.

An Example of a Weight Loss Meal Plan Consisting of 1,200 Calories per Week

Day 1: The Morning Meal

In a dish, combine three-quarters of a cup of bran flakes, one banana, and one cup of fat-free milk.

Lunch

To make a pita sandwich, take one small whole wheat pita, three ounces of turkey breast, half of the roasted pepper, one teaspoon of mayonnaise, and lettuce leaves and place them in a sandwich maker. Serve with one stick of string cheese made from part-skim mozzarella and two kiwis.

Dinner

Serve 4 ounces of broiled flounder or sole with 2 plum tomatoes cut thinly and topped with 2 tablespoons of grated Parmesan cheese. Broil the tomatoes until they are barely golden brown. Serve with one cup of couscous that has been cooked and one cup of steamed broccoli. Dessert should consist of a single serving of ice cream, please.

Breakfast On the Second Day

Create a smoothie by combining one cup of frozen berries, one-half of a banana, and eight ounces of low-fat or fat-free milk. Grab one or two eggs that have been hard-boiled on your way out the door.

Day 2: Lunch

Warm up one cup of vegetarian vegetable soup and serve it with one veggie burger on top of a piece of toast made with healthy grains and seeds or an English muffin. To complete the dish, add one cup of fresh grapes.

Day 2: Dinner

Brush 4 ounces of boneless, skinless chicken breast with barbecue sauce and grill. Add some chopped scallions and a squeeze of lime juice to the chicken before serving. Serve with one half of a simple baked or sweet potato and two heaping cups of spinach that have been sautéed. Garlic, olive oil, and tomatoes should also be used in this dish.

Breakfast On Day Three

In the microwave, heat 1/2 cup of quick-cooking oats with low-fat or unsweetened soy milk. Add 1/2 apple (sliced or diced), 1 teaspoon of honey, and a sprinkle of cinnamon.

Day 3: Lunch

To prepare a chicken salad, combine 4 ounces of shredded skinless roast chicken breast with 1/4 cup sliced red grapes, 1 tablespoon slivered almonds or nuts of choice, 1/4 cup chopped celery, 1 tablespoon mayonnaise, and 1 tablespoon plain, unsweetened Greek yogurt. Serve over lettuce. Eat with 1 big slice of multigrain bread.

Day 3: Dinner

In addition to 3 cups of steamed spinach, serve 4 ounces of steamed shrimp, one baked potato topped with 3 tablespoons of salsa and one tablespoon of unsweetened Greek yogurt, and one baked potato. To finish off the meal, have an ounce of chocolate or an ice cream bar that has between 100 and 150 calories.

Breakfast On the Fourth Day

To create a simple yet scrumptious yogurt parfait, layer one cup of plain or low-sugar Greek yogurt on top of one cup of your preferred berries and one-third cup of sugar-free granola.

Day 4: Lunch

Warm up one cup of tomato soup and serve it with a sandwich that consists of one tiny pita prepared with whole wheat, three ounces of thinly sliced roast beef, one teaspoon of horseradish, mustard, tomato slices, and lettuce. Consume two cups of raw vegetables and one-fourth cup of hummus.

Day 4: Dinner

Poach 4 ounces of salmon and prepare a slaw by combining 1 1/4 cups of coleslaw mix, 2 sliced scallions, 1 tablespoon of rice vinegar, and 1 1/2 teaspoons of olive oil together. Serve the salad with the fish. To taste, add various seasonings, spices, and herbs. Combine with one cup of a grain that is 100% whole, such as quinoa.

Breakfast On the Fifth Day

In a bowl, mix together 6 ounces of plain, unsweetened Greek yogurt, one cup of Cheerios, one-half cup of berries, and one tablespoon of slivered almonds, and the mixture should be Cheerios.

Day 5: Lunch

To make a quesadilla, spread one-fourth of a cup of fat-free refried beans over a tortilla made of maize that has been stone-ground. 1 ounce of shredded part-skim cheese should be sprinkled on top. Place another tortilla on top of the salsa, then either microwave it for 45 seconds on high or grill it. Cucumber spears, a half cup of cottage cheese or Greek yogurt with 2% fat, and two clementines should be served with this dish.

Day 5: Dinner

3 ounces of roasted pork tenderloin should be served with 1 cup of baked acorn squash that has been mashed with a pinch of cinnamon. Two to three cups of salad greens

should be served with a dash of olive oil and as much vinegar as desired. For dessert, you can serve chocolate or a bar of ice cream that has between 100 and 150 calories.

Breakfast On the Sixth Day

A 100% whole-grain frozen waffle should be toasted, and then two teaspoons of nut butter should be put on top. Include one tiny sliced banana, as well as ground cinnamon and nutmeg, in the recipe. To serve, pour eight ounces of fat-free milk over the top.

Day 6: Lunch

To make a tuna pita, you will need one tiny whole-wheat pita, two ounces of tuna that have been packed in water, and one tablespoon of mayonnaise, mustard, cucumber, and onion slices. Serve with ten tiny carrots, three-quarters of a cup of Greek yogurt that is plain and unsweetened, and a small pear.

Day 6: Dinner

To make jambalaya, combine 3/4 cup cooked brown rice with 1/2 cup corn, 2 ounces cooked sliced turkey sausage, 1/3 cup salsa, and 1/4 cup salt-free black or navy beans in a saucepan and heat over medium-high heat until everything is well combined and heated through. Eat with three cups of spinach and garlic that have been sautéed in one tablespoon of olive oil.

Day 7: For breakfast, layer one ounce of reduced-fat sliced cheese, one tomato slice, one cup of steamed and drained spinach, and one poached egg on half of an English muffin that has been toasted. Accompany each serving with a grapefruit.

Day 7: Lunch

To make black bean salad, combine one-half cup of chopped red bell peppers, one-half cup of orange slices, one-half cup of canned black beans, one-half cup of scallions, one teaspoon of vinegar, and one-half cup of canned black beans. Place on top of salad greens and serve with one tortilla made from stone-ground corn 100 percent and a piece of fruit on the side.

Day 7: Dinner

Serve 3 ounces of broiled or grilled flank steak with one baked sweet potato with 1 teaspoon of butter, 1 cup of steamed zucchini, and 1 1/2 cups of berries.

Grocery Shopping

Going to the grocery store is one of the many critical steps involved in selecting nutritious foods to eat. When going grocery shopping, it's vital to put the majority of your attention on selecting nutrient-dense, whole foods like fruits, vegetables, lean proteins, and grains that are unprocessed.

Additionally, it is essential to refrain from buying processed meals and junk food since these types of foods often have a large number of calories, sugar, and fats that are undesirable for you. Instead, put your attention on stocking up on complete, healthy meals that will help you achieve your weight reduction objectives.

Eating Out: When it comes to picking nutritious meal selections, dining out may be a difficult challenge. You may, however, continue to enjoy dining out while adhering to a healthy diet so long as you pay attention to the sizes of the portions you order and choose appropriate selections.

When dining out, some helpful suggestions include going for selections that are grilled or baked, going for salads, and staying away from condiments that are high in calories, such as mayonnaise and cheese. You will be able to keep your weight reduction program on track and continue to make progress toward your objectives if you choose healthy meal options when you dine out.

Incorporating Exercise into Your Everyday Routine

A key element of a healthy lifestyle is making movement a regular part of one's routine since this helps maintain a healthy weight. Finding activities that you love, making goals that are attainable, and keeping track of your progress are just a few of the suggestions and tactics that we will discuss in this subchapter about the topic of integrating more physical exercise into your day-to-day routine.

Finding Activities, You Enjoy

Finding things that you love is an essential step in the process of introducing physical exercise into your daily routine. Finding activities that you enjoy is important. If you choose things that you love doing, you will have a better chance of continuing to do them and incorporating physical exercise into your daily routine.

Hiking, cycling, yoga, and dancing are all possible pastimes that might appeal to your sense of adventure. Make sure that any physical exercise you decide to include in your daily routine is one that you take pleasure in and that you look forward to doing so.

Setting Achievable Goals

Establishing objectives that are within your reach Establishing goals that are within your reach is another essential component of including physical exercise in your daily routine. You may prevent feelings of discouragement and overload as well as keep yourself motivated and focused on your work if you establish objectives that are within your reach. It is vital to begin goal-setting with a modest ambition and to progressively raise the difficulty and intensity of your exercises as you go toward achieving those objectives. For instance, if you are not used to engaging in physical activity, you should begin by doing mild exercise for ten to fifteen minutes every day. As you get more experienced, you should progressively extend the duration of your workouts and raise the difficulty level.

Keeping tabs on your advancement

Maintaining your motivation and staying focused on your objectives is much easier when you keep track of your progress. You may get a better idea of how far you've gone and where you still have room for improvement if you keep track of your progress. As you continue to include physical exercise into your daily routine, this may assist you in maintaining your concentration and motivation levels.

Keeping a fitness diary, utilizing a fitness app, or documenting your exercises on a calendar are all viable options for monitoring your improvement as you work toward your fitness goals. Pick the strategy that delivers the greatest outcomes for you, then commit to using it consistently so that you may appreciate the fruits of your labor and commitment.

Taking on More Healthful Practices

The development of healthy routines is another important aspect of a lifestyle that is conducive to weight loss. In this subchapter, we will study several recommendations and tactics for adopting healthy habits, such as getting enough sleep, minimizing stress, and keeping hydrated. Among the other topics that we will cover in this subchapter are:

Adequate Amount of Sleep

Obtaining an adequate amount of sleep is essential to get an adequate amount of sleep-in order to keep a healthy weight and ensure general well-being. If you don't get enough sleep, your body will create more of the hormone cortisol, which has been shown to stimulate hunger and contribute to unhealthy levels of food consumption.

It is advised that you receive between seven and nine hours of sleep every night in order to assist in the regulation of your hormones and to promote a healthy weight. In addition, the development of a regular nighttime ritual and the creation of an atmosphere that is favorable to sleep are both helpful in enhancing the quality of one's slumber.

Getting Rid of Stress

Lessening one's exposure to stress is yet another crucial component of developing healthy practices. If you're under a lot of pressure, your body will create more of the hormone cortisol, which has been shown to stimulate hunger and contribute to unhealthy levels of food consumption.

Exercising, practicing mindfulness meditation, and spending time with loved ones are just a few of the numerous activities that might help relieve stress. Choose the techniques that help you feel the most relaxed, and make it a point to prioritize stress reduction in your day-to-day activities.

Maintaining An Adequate Water Intake

Maintaining an adequate water intake is essential for maintaining a healthy weight as well as one's general health and well-being. If you are dehydrated, your body may confuse thirst with hunger, which may cause you to consume more food than you need.

In order to maintain proper hydration levels throughout the day, it is advised that at least eight glasses of water be consumed. Incorporating additional hydrating drinks, such as herbal tea, into your daily routine will also assist you in maintaining proper hydration and provide support for your efforts to achieve your weight reduction objectives.

In conclusion, selecting nutritious foods to eat, adding physical exercise into your daily routine, and developing healthy behaviors are all components of a lifestyle that is conducive to maintaining a healthy weight. You will be able to make long-lasting changes to your lifestyle and accomplish your weight reduction objectives if you read this chapter and follow the guidelines and advice that are presented in it. Keep in mind that achieving success does not happen overnight, but if you are persistent, dedicated, and have a positive mentality, you may accomplish your objectives and experience a transformation in both your body and your life.

CHAPTER 4

Staying Motivated and On Track

When it comes to getting rid of excess weight, maintaining motivation and keeping on track are two of the most difficult obstacles. In this chapter, we will discuss a variety of suggestions and techniques for maintaining your motivation and keeping on track with your goal to lose weight.

Establishing Objectives That Can Be Met

One of the keys to being motivated and on track is setting objectives that are really attainable. You are putting yourself in a position to fail by establishing objectives that are either too unrealistic or too ambitious for you to achieve, and this may lead to feelings of frustration and a loss of drive.

When determining what you want to accomplish, it is vital to take into account a variety of characteristics, including your age, height, present weight, and degree of physical activity. Setting both short-term and long-term objectives is essential if you want to ensure that you have something to work for in the here and now as well as in the future.

Recognizing and Honoring Your Achievements

One further essential part of maintaining your motivation and keeping on track is to have regular celebrations of your achievements. When you reward your efforts and commitment by celebrating your accomplishments, you keep yourself motivated and focused by recognizing the value of your hard work.

There are various methods to recognize and celebrate your achievements, including purchasing yourself a reward, indulging in a day at the spa, or just making the effort to reflect on and appreciate your achievements. Pick the approaches that suit you the most, and make it a point to honor each milestone along the way as you embark on your road to a healthier weight.

Putting Yourself in a Position to Be Supported

Keeping oneself motivated and on track requires a number of crucial components, one of which is surrounding yourself with support. When you have support, you have those who will encourage you and keep you accountable, which increases the likelihood that you will continue to be motivated and on track.

There are many different methods to surround oneself with support, such as becoming a member of a weight loss support group, maintaining relationships with friends and family, or engaging the services of a personal trainer. Pick the approaches that suit you the most, and make it a goal to surround yourself with people who will encourage you on your quest to a healthier weight.

Keeping Oneself Accountable

Keeping oneself responsible is another essential part of maintaining one's motivation and keeping on track. Because you feel responsible to both yourself and the people around you when you keep accountable, you are more likely to continue working toward the objectives you have set for yourself and to achieve progress.

Keeping a food journal, keeping track of your exercises, or engaging with a coach or a mentor are just some of the numerous ways that you may ensure that you are held responsible. Pick the approaches that suit you the most, and make it a top priority to hold yourself responsible while you're on your path to losing weight.

Determine Why You Want to Lose Weight

Keeping yourself motivated and on track during your quest to lose weight is also essential to your overall success. You can maintain your motivation and remain on track to accomplish your weight reduction objectives if you establish goals that are within your reach, celebrate your successes as you go, surround yourself with people who will encourage you, and hold yourself responsible. Keep in mind that achieving success does not happen overnight, but if you are persistent, dedicated, and have a positive mentality, you may accomplish your objectives and experience a transformation in both your body and your life.

Find out the Reasons Behind Your Obsession with Weight Loss

Write down all of the reasons you want to lose weight and make sure they are clear in your mind. This will help you maintain your commitment to your weight reduction objectives and keep you encouraged along the way. Make it a habit to go through them on a regular basis and consult them whenever you feel tempted to deviate from the path you've set out to take to lose weight. You could want to lose weight to reduce your risk of developing diabetes, so you can keep up with your grandkids so that you can look your best at an event so that you can improve your self-confidence, or so that you can wear a certain pair of pants.

Think and speak in a constructive manner.

People who have optimistic expectations and who are confident in their capacity to accomplish their objectives often have more success in their weight loss efforts. Additionally, those who engage in "change discussion" have a higher probability of carrying out their goals. Talking about change is making declarations about one's commitment to making behavioral changes, the motivations driving those changes, and the actions that will be taken or are being taken to achieve one's objectives.

Therefore, you should immediately begin having optimistic conversations regarding your weight reduction. In addition to this, verbalize the actions that you want to carry out, and commit your ideas to paper. On the other hand, studies have shown that individuals who devote a significant portion of their time to daydreaming just about their ideal weight are less likely to achieve their objective. This practice is known as psychologically indulging oneself. Contrast is what you should be doing in your mind instead. Spend a few minutes seeing yourself achieving your target weight, and then spend another few minutes visualizing any potential roadblocks that may stand in your way on the path there. This will help you mentally contrast the two scenarios.

A group of 134 students participated in research in which they were asked to either mentally indulge or mentally contrast their dieting objectives. Those who were able to mentally contrast the two options were more inclined to act. They increased the amount of physical activity they did in addition to reducing the number of high-calorie items they consumed. According to the findings of this study, mentally contrasting is more effective at motivating people to take action and leads to more action than mentally indulging. Mental indulging can lead your brain to believe that you have already achieved your goals, which can prevent you from ever taking any action to achieve them.

Don't Strive for Perfection, and Be Sure to Forgive Yourself When You Fall Short

To reduce weight, you do not need to be flawless in any way. If you take an "all or nothing" attitude to achieving your objectives, you will have a lower chance of doing so. If you place too many limitations on yourself, you can find yourself thinking things like, "I had a hamburger and fries for lunch, so I might as well have pizza for supper." Try to phrase it like, "I had a huge lunch; therefore, I should strive for a healthy supper." This will seem much more natural. Also, try not to be too hard on yourself when you do something wrong. Your motivation will suffer if you dwell on negative ideas about yourself. Instead, extend mercy to yourself. Keep in mind that making just one mistake will not derail all of your hard work.

Acquire a healthy love and appreciation for your physical form.

Researchers have discovered time and time again that those who loathe their bodies are less inclined to make an effort to reduce their weight. Taking action to enhance your body image may help you lose more weight and keep it off in the long run. People who have a more positive perception of their bodies are also more inclined to choose a diet that they can stick to and experiment with new activities that will assist them in accomplishing their objectives.

The Following Activities May Help You Have a Better Perception of Your Body

- Do something for yourself, like getting a massage or manicure
- Surround yourself with positive people
- Stop comparing yourself to others, especially models
- Wear clothes that you like and that fit well
- Look in the mirror and say the things you like about yourself out loud
- Exercise
- Appreciate what your body can do
- Do something for yourself
- Surround yourself with positive people
- Stop comparing yourself to others, especially models
- Wear clothes that you like and that fit well
- Look in the mirror and say the things you like about yourself out loud.

Find A Role Model

If you want to remain motivated to lose weight, having a role model to look up to might assist. Nevertheless, in order to keep oneself motivated; you need to choose the appropriate sort of role model. You will not be motivated in the long run by just pinning a photo of a supermodel on your refrigerator. Instead, look for a person that may readily serve as a model for you to emulate and connect to. You could find it easier to maintain your motivation if you have a good role model who is also relatable. Perhaps you have a buddy who has successfully battled their weight and can serve as a source of motivation for you. You might also browse motivational tales or blogs written by individuals who have successfully lost weight and share their experiences.

Obtain a Dog.

It's been shown that having a dog at your side may help you lose weight. In point of fact, several studies have shown that having a dog helps facilitate weight loss for its owners. To begin, having a dog might encourage you to move around more. According to the findings of research conducted in Canada on dog owners, those who had dogs walked for an average of 300 minutes per week, but those who did not have dogs walked for just 168 minutes on average each week. Second, dogs are wonderful sources of emotional and social support. Dogs, in contrast to your human workout partner, will nearly always be happy to participate in some kind of physical exercise.

Getting Past Obstacles & Obstacle Courses

During the course of your quest to lose weight, it is certain that you may run across roadblocks and difficulties along the path. It is essential to have a strategy for conquering these obstacles and problems in order to maintain your motivation and continue moving forward with your plans.

It is crucial to reevaluate both your objectives and your methods after experiencing a setback so that you may more effectively go forward. It's possible that you need to make some alterations to the objectives you have set for yourself or switch up the technique you're taking. It is also essential to treat oneself with kindness and refrain from having critical conversations with yourself since doing so might cause a loss of drive.

Maintaining One's Concentration While Being Steadfast

One other essential component of keeping oneself motivated and on the course is to maintain one's concentration and consistency. It is far more probable that you will advance toward your objectives and realize them if you maintain your concentration and remain constant.

Keeping your objectives at the forefront of your mind is one strategy that might help you maintain your focus and consistency. Put your objectives in writing and display them in a place where you can see them to serve as a constant reminder of what it is you are striving to achieve. Having a plan that you follow, even on the days when you don't feel like it, is one more approach to maintaining your concentration and consistency in your actions.

Adopting a Mentality of Continuous Improvement

The adoption of a development mindset is another essential component in maintaining one's motivation and staying on course. If you have a growth mindset, you feel that you have the capacity to develop and improve and that failures and difficulties are chances for you to grow and learn from your experiences.

When you have a growth mindset, you are less likely to regard failures and setbacks as defeats and more likely to view them as chances for development and learning. This makes it easier for you to remain motivated and on track with your goals. This frame of mind may assist you in maintaining your motivation and staying on track, even on the days that are the most challenging.

CHAPTER 5

Maintaining Your Lean Lifestyle for Long-Term Success

In the last chapter of "The Slim Mindset: Transform Your Body and Life with Sustainable Weight Loss," we will discuss how to keep your lean lifestyle going for a long time and how this will contribute to your success in the long run. Even if achieving your desired weight and reshaping your body is a vital objective, it is of equal significance to ensure that you will be able to maintain these changes over the long term.

Recognizing the Importance of Preventative Maintenance

Recognizing the significance of maintenance as a first step in ensuring your success in leading a leaner lifestyle over the long run is essential. Altering your eating and exercise routines in a way that is both healthy and sustainable for the long term is the focus of a lean lifestyle, in contrast to conventional diets, which often result in rapid weight loss followed by an equally rapid return to previous weight levels.

In order to successfully control one's weight, one must first adopt a healthy lifestyle. This means gaining information about diet and exercise, maintaining a good attitude, and being motivated in the appropriate way. Your chances of achieving successful weight management for the rest of your life are improved when you are driven from the inside out by goals such as improved health, more energy, higher self-esteem, and greater personal control.

Always keep in mind that your objectives should be attainable, and keep your focus on the long term. If you have faith in yourself, you will succeed. The information that is shown here will provide you with suggestions that will assist you in achieving the objectives that you have set.

Control Your Home Environment

- You are only allowed to consume food when seated at the kitchen or dining room table.
- Do not eat while doing other activities such as watching television, reading, cooking, chatting on

the phone, working at the computer, or standing in front of the refrigerator.

- Don't bring enticing meals into the home, and don't purchase them either.

- Hide all of the foods that might entice you. Have quick access to meals that are low in calories.

- If you are not currently making a meal, you are not permitted in the kitchen.

- Always have a selection of nutritious snacks available to you, including bite-sized pieces of fruit and vegetables, fruit in cans, pretzels, low-fat string cheese, and nonfat cottage cheese.

Take charge of your working conditions.

o Do not eat at your work or have enticing treats at your desk.

o If you find that you are becoming hungry in between meals, you should prepare some nutritious snacks and carry them with you to the office.

- o   Instead of eating during your breaks, you could go for a stroll instead.

- o   If your job involves dealing with food in any way, you should prepare the one thing you will consume at mealtimes in advance.

- o   Make it difficult for yourself to pick at food by chewing gum, sugar-free candies, or sipping water or another liquid low in calories while you are in the same room.

- o   You should not continue to work through meals. If you skip meals, your metabolism will slow down, which might lead to you eating too much at the following meal.

- o   If food is served for special occasions, choose the healthiest choice, munch on low-fat snacks brought from home, choose one option and have a tiny quantity of it, choose not to have anything, select one option and have just a beverage, or choose not to have anything at all.

Control Your Mealtime Environment

- o Place your dish of food on the burner or the counter in the kitchen to serve it. It is imperative that the serving plates not be placed on the table. If you choose to place dishes on the table, remember to take them away as soon as you are through eating.

- o On your plate, put half of it dedicated to vegetables, a quarter of it to lean proteins, and the remaining quarter to starches.

- o Utilize dishes, bowls, and glasses that are on the smaller side. When placed in a tiny dish, a piece that is really on the smaller side will seem to be much larger.

- o Please be courteous and decline further help.

- o When arranging the food on your plate, keep quantities to no more than one scoop or dish at a time.

Management of One's Daily Diet

- If you want to break your association with eating, choose another thing to do instead of eating.

- Hold off on satisfying your urge for anything to eat for twenty minutes.

- Before you start eating, be sure you down a full glass of water or diet Coke.

- Throughout the day, be sure to sip from a large glass or bottle of water that you have handy.

- Steer clear of condiments and add-ons that are rich in calories, such as cream for your coffee, butter, mayonnaise, and salad dressings.

Shopping

- Shopping should not be done while you are hungry or weary.

- When you go shopping, bring a list with you, and don't purchase anything that's not on the list.

- If you really have to indulge in enticing foods, purchase them in smaller portions and look for alternatives that are fewer in calories.

- Do not try out different flavors when shopping.

- Make sure you read the labels on your food. Compare different items so that you may choose the ones that are best for your health.

Preparing

- In The Meanwhile, Prepare Your Food While Chewing on A Piece of Gum.

- If you want to test the flavor of your dish, use a quarter of a teaspoon.

- Make every effort to prepare just the amount of food that you want to consume, so eliminating any possibility of eating more.

- If you have made more food than you need, divide it up into separate containers, and either freeze it or put it in the refrigerator as soon as possible.

- Refrain from eating snacks while you are preparing meals.

Consumption

- Take your time eating.

- Keep in mind that it takes around twenty minutes for your stomach to signal to your brain that it has reached its capacity for food.

- Don't allow a lack of real hunger to trick you into thinking you need more food.

- The best method to eat is to start by taking a bite, putting down your fork, drinking a sip of water, cutting your next bite, taking a little, putting down your utensil, and continuing in this manner until you have completed your meal.

- Do not attempt to cut all of your food at once. Only make cuts when necessary.

- Chew your meal thoroughly and eat in manageable chunks.

- At least once throughout a meal or snack, take a break from eating, even if it's only for a minute or two. Take some time out of your day to relax, think, and talk to someone.

Disposal of Waste and Remaining Food

• Clearly label any leftovers that will be used for a certain meal or snack.

• Freeze or freeze leftovers in their separate pieces, and then use them as needed.

• If you are still hungry, you should not clean up the mess.

Consuming Meals in Public and Eating with Others

- Do not show up for the meeting hungry.
- Consume something rather light before dinner.
- Make an effort to satiate yourself with meals that are low in calories, such as vegetables and fruit, and limit yourself to smaller amounts of foods that are high in calories.
- Consume the foods you like, but limit yourself to smaller quantities.
- Whether you want seconds, wait at least twenty minutes after you have finished eating to see if you are genuinely hungry or if your eyes are larger than your stomach. This will help you choose whether or not you should give in to your cravings.
- Reduce your use of alcoholic drinks. You could try some soda water with a slice of lime in it.

- Refrain from skipping any other meals during the day in order to conserve your stomach space for the important occasion.

At Restaurants

• Order a la carte rather than buffet style.
Instead of eating bread as an appetizer, you could consider ordering some veggies or a salad.

• If you order a meal that is rich in calories, split it with a friend or family member.

• If you want something refreshing after supper, try a mint with your coffee. If you do decide to eat dessert, be sure you split it with at least two other individuals.

• Eat just until you are satisfied; if you overeat, you will end up wasting food. In order to take additional food home with you, ask for a doggy bag.

• Before the waiter brings you the rest of the meal, give them the instruction to pack up half of your dinner in a takeout container.

• Make sure to request high-fat condiments like salad dressing, gravy, and sauces on the side. Before you take each mouthful, dip the very tip of your fork in the dressing.

• If there is bread available, you should only request one slice of it. You should try it without butter or oil first. In Italian restaurants where oil and vinegar are offered with bread, the proper way to dip the bread is with very little oil and a significant quantity of vinegar.

When Attending the Home of a Friend

- Make an Offer to Bring a Dish, Appetizer, or Dessert That Is Lower in Calories
- Either serve yourself a tiny bit or communicate to the host that you only want a little portion of whatever they are serving.
- Please move away from the snack table and either stand or sit there. Keep your distance from the kitchen, and if you must be there, keep yourself occupied.

Reduce the amount of alcohol you drink.

Wherever there are Buffets or Cafeterias

• Make sure that lettuce and/or vegetables take up the majority of the space on your plate.

• Instead of a dinner dish, you should use a salad plate.

• After you've finished dining, clean the table before getting a cup of coffee or tea.

Hosting Get-Togethers at Your Place

• Look into several cookbooks that are low in fat and cholesterol.

• opt for things that are already portioned out, such as chicken breasts or hamburger patties.

• Make appetizers and sweets that are lower in calories.

Holidays

• Hide all of the foods that might entice you.

• Stay away from edible items while decorating the home.

• Ensure that visitors have access to low-calorie drinks and snacks throughout their stay.

• Permit yourself one well-considered reward every day.

• Refrain from skipping meals in order to store up more calories for the festive supper. Consume your food in accordance with a schedule.

Exercise Well

• Make getting regular exercise a top priority and schedule it into your day.

• If at all feasible, walk the full or at least a portion of the distance to your place of employment.

• Find a friend to work out with you. You may go to the gym, run or walk with a buddy, or stroll around the mall with a shopping partner during one of your breaks. You could even go for a walk with a coworker during one of your breaks.

• Park your vehicle in the very back of the parking lot, and then walk to the front door of the shop or office.

• You should always use the stairs to go to your floor, either all the way or at least part of the way.

• If you work at a desk, get up and move about the office at regular intervals.

• While you are seated at your workstation, raise your legs up and down.

• Spend your weekends doing something active outdoors, like going on a walk or a bike ride, for example.

Maintain a Positive Mental Attitude

• Make your health a top priority when it comes to weight control.

• Be practical. Set as your objective the improvement of your health rather than achieving the lowest possible weight or the optimum weight determined by calculations or charts.

• Instead of focusing on dieting, make adopting good eating habits your first priority. Dieting is often only successful for a limited period of time and seldom leads to sustainable weight loss.

• Focus on the long term. You are in the process of building new healthy habits that you will continue to follow in the next month, in the following year, and in the following decade.

Making Adjustments as Needed

It's possible that as you go farther along in your quest to lose weight, your priorities and requirements may shift. It is vital to make modifications to your diet and exercise routine as necessary in order to ensure that you are still on track to attain your objectives and sustain the success that you have made.

Shedding pounds

Shedding pounds is not a process that unfolds in a straight line over time. If you reduce the number of calories you consume, you may shed some weight in the first few weeks, but after that, something could change. You don't change the number of calories that you consume, yet you notice that your weight loss is slower or perhaps stops altogether. This is due to the fact that when you lose weight, in addition to reducing fat, you also lose water and lean tissue. Additionally, your metabolism will slow down, and your body will alter in other ways. Therefore, if you want to continue losing weight each week, you need to continue decreasing the number of calories you consume

A Calorie Isn't Usually a Calorie

There are many different things that may contain a calorie. Consuming 100 calories worth of broccoli, for instance, might have a very different impact on your body in comparison to consuming 100 calories worth of high-fructose corn syrup. The key to successful long-term weight reduction is to give up eating items like candies that are high in calories but don't make you feel full, and to switch to eating meals that are satisfying without being high in calories, such as vegetables, fish, and whole grains (like vegetables).

Many Of Us Don't Always Eat to Satisfy the Hunger

A good number of us don't always eat for the sole purpose of satiating our hunger. We also resort to eating for comfort or to alleviate stress, which is another reason why any strategy to lose weight may soon go off the rails.

Cut carbohydrates

A fresh perspective on the battle against obesity sees the issue as not being one of ingesting an excessive number of calories, but rather the manner in which fat is accumulated in the body as a result of eating carbs, namely the function that the hormone insulin plays in this process. When you consume a meal, the glucose that comes from the carbohydrate content of the food enters your circulation. Your body will always metabolize the glucose from a meal first before it moves on to the fat, and this is done so that your blood sugar levels may be maintained at a healthy level.

When you consume a meal that is high in carbohydrates (such as a lot of pasta, rice, bread, or French fries, for example), your body will secrete insulin in order to assist with the rapid increase in the amount of glucose that is present in your blood. Insulin blocks your fat cells from releasing fat for the body to burn as fuel (since its goal is to burn off glucose), and it makes additional fat cells for storing anything that your body can't burn off. In addition to managing blood sugar levels, insulin performs these two functions. The end effect is that you put on weight, and since your body needs more fuel to burn, you consume more food to satisfy that need. You have a need for carbohydrates since insulin is only able to burn them, which starts a vicious cycle in which you consume carbohydrates and gain weight. According to this line of thinking, in order to lose weight, you need to interrupt this cycle by limiting the number of carbohydrates you eat.

Cut fat

If you don't want to gain weight, you shouldn't consume fat, since this is a fundamental principle of many different eating plans. If you go down any aisle at a grocery store, you will be inundated with options for low-fat snacks, dairy products, and pre-packaged meals. But at the same time as low-fat food alternatives have proliferated, the prevalence of obesity has skyrocketed. Therefore, why haven't more of us found success with low-fat diets?

1. Not all kinds of fat are unhealthy. Fats that are healthy for you, often known as "good" fats, may really aid in weight control, mood management, and the battle against weariness. Avocados, nuts, seeds, soy milk, tofu, and fatty fish all contain a type of fat called unsaturated fat, which helps you feel fuller for longer. Adding a little bit of flavorful olive oil to a plate of vegetables, for example, can make it easier to eat healthy food and improve the overall quality of your diet.

2. We often choose the incorrect path when faced with a choice. A significant number of us make the error of replacing the calories we get from fat with the calories we get from sugar and processed carbs. For instance, rather than consuming full-fat yogurt, we consume variants of yogurt that are lower in fat or have no fat at all but are loaded with sugar to make up for the diminished flavor. Or, instead of having a fatty breakfast item like bacon, we choose something like a doughnut or muffin, which promotes quick increases in blood sugar.

Keeping Yourself Current with New Information

When it comes to keeping your slim lifestyle for the long term, one of the most essential things you can do is to educate yourself on good eating and exercise practices. This could entail reading books, going to seminars, or seeing a professional nutritionist or personal trainer for guidance.

Ignorance is never a valid reason for anything. After all, we are the product of the food that we consume, and the widespread ignorance of nutrition continues to astound me. Every piece of food that you put in your mouth has an effect, not only on the amount of fat you lose and how your body looks to others, but also on your overall health, and this effect may be deep and can endure for a very long time. When it comes to obtaining results in the real world, the fact that I include guidance on nutrition and supplements as an essential component of all of our personal training recommendations has served me very well.

It is essential that you educate yourself on how to lose weight. This entails engaging in activities such as reading books and viewing films, conversing with others who have personally gone through the experience, and seeking the advice of an expert. If you have the right knowledge, you'll be able to make more informed choices regarding the kinds of foods to eat, the amount of physical activity you should get, and the number of calories you should take in on a daily basis.

In addition to this, having an understanding of how your body functions can assist you in comprehending the factors that contribute to your slower-than-desired weight loss. If you know, for instance, that consuming carbs causes an increase in insulin levels, this knowledge may help you make more informed decisions about the foods you put into your body.

Introducing Variation into Your Everyday Activities

Adding a little bit of diversity to your daily activities might help you stay motivated and stop boredom from creeping in before it ever starts. To maintain a sense of novelty and interest in your routine, experiment with different forms of exercise, try out new recipes, and look into other ways of eating healthfully.

Keeping Yourself Responsible and Accountable

Last but not least, if you want your healthy lifestyle to be sustainable over the long run, you need to be responsible for yourself. This entails being truthful with yourself on your progress, keeping a log of your eating and exercise routines, and modifying those routines as necessary.

CONCLUSION

The book "The Lean Mindset: Transform Your Body and Life with Sustainable Weight Loss" provides a thorough guide to assist you in achieving your weight loss goals in a manner that is both healthy and sustainable. You may effect a change in both your body and your life that will be long-lasting if you take on a lean mentality and put the concepts and techniques that are discussed in this book into practice.

In the first chapter, we spoke about how important it is to have a growth-oriented mindset when it comes to losing weight and understanding your body. In the previous chapter, "Chapter 2: Strategies for Changing Your Mentality and Overcoming Common Obstacles," we discussed many methods for altering one's mindset and overcoming various impediments that may be preventing one from

In chapter 3, we examined the adoption of a lean lifestyle, including advice for healthy food, effective exercise, and stress management. This chapter also included a discussion on how to handle stress. In addition to this, we went through the significance of establishing a schedule for yourself that is not only effective but also durable.

In chapter 4, we discussed the several methods that may be used to keep oneself motivated and on track, such as establishing objectives that are attainable, keeping track of one's progress, and getting support from friends and family. Finally, in chapter 5, we covered the necessity of sustaining your healthy lifestyle for long-term success. This included developing a support system, recognizing your victories, remaining focused on your objectives, and continuing to educate yourself.

You will be able to establish a healthy lifestyle that is not only practical but also long-lasting if you read this book and put the advice and suggestions it contains into practice. You may reach your weight reduction objectives and improve both your body and your life in a manner that is sustainable if you are persistent, dedicated, and have a good mental attitude.

In a nutshell, the secret to long-term, healthy weight reduction is not in just decreasing one's caloric intake or adhering to a regimented eating strategy, but rather in embracing new habits of thought and behavior. Having a "lean mentality" means adopting a "holistic approach to health and wellbeing," which means incorporating good behaviors into your everyday life in a manner that is both sustainable and pleasurable. This is at the heart of the "lean mindset."

It is essential to keep in mind that losing weight is not a one-time occurrence but rather a process that occurs over the course of a trip. You will run across obstacles along the road, but if you have the appropriate strategies, resources, and mentality, you will be able to overcome those obstacles and accomplish what you set out to do.

It is up to you to put these ideas and strategies into action and incorporate them into your life in order to build a solid foundation for achievement, which is provided by the concepts and methods described in this book. You won't believe how soon you will get results if you start off slowly and steadily increasing your efforts. In addition, as you continue to make improvements, you will acquire the self-assurance, expertise, and routines that are necessary for your long-term success.

Consequently, you should adopt the concept of lean living and take the first step toward improving both your body and your life. You may reach your weight reduction objectives and live a life that is healthier, happier, and more rewarding if you are persistent, dedicated, and have a good attitude throughout the process.

It is essential to keep in mind that shedding extra pounds is a personal journey, and the specifics of that trip will vary from person to person. Try not to judge yourself too harshly or compare yourself unfavorably to others. Honor your victories, but don't forget to draw lessons from your defeats. Most essential, remember to have patience. Losing weight is not a fast cure, but rather an ongoing commitment to improving one's health and well-being.

Reach out to loved ones, friends, or a trained counselor if you feel as if you may use some assistance along the journey. Put yourself in an environment where you're always surrounded by upbeat, encouraging, and supporting individuals. Also, if you have any worries or questions, you should never be afraid to see a medical professional.

In conclusion, "The Lean Mindset: Improve Your Body and Life with Sustainable Weight Loss" gives you access to the skills, resources, and direction you need to reach your weight loss objectives and transform both your body and your life in a manner that is both healthy and sustainable.

You have the ability to lead a life that is happier, healthier, and more meaningful if you adopt the appropriate mentality, behaviors, and network of support. Therefore, make the first move now and get started on your road to a healthier, more energized version of yourself.